Distribution, publication, and copying in any form are prohibited and subject to damages.

TEN HYPNOSES

Copying, publishing, and sharing with third parties are only permitted with the written consent of the author. Please observe the notes on copyright and usage.

Distribution, publication, and copying in any form are prohibited and subject to damages.

Copying, publishing, and sharing with third parties are only permitted with the written consent of the author. Please observe the notes on copyright and usage.

Distribution, publication, and copying in any form are prohibited and subject to damages.

Ingo Michael Simon

TEN HYPNOSES

25
FEAR IN CROWDS, AGORAPHOBIA

Copying, publishing, and sharing with third parties are only permitted with the written consent of the author. Please observe the notes on copyright and usage.

Distribution, publication, and copying in any form are prohibited and subject to damages.

© 2024 Ingo Michael Simon
All rights reserved.
Independently published
www.ingosimon.com

Important Notes for Urgent Attention:
The contents of this book are based on the practical experiences of the author with hypnosis applications and psychotherapy in a trance state. Although the author has strived for the utmost care, errors or misunderstandings in the presentation cannot be completely excluded. Therapeutic work with people and the application of hypnosis are solely the responsibility of the hypnotist. It cannot be ruled out that parts of this book may be misunderstood or that the application of a presented procedure may cause an undesirable reaction in the client. The author also assumes no co-responsibility if work with a client is carried out with reference to the statements in this book.

The Author:
Ingo Michael Simon studied psychology and education and is a hypnotherapist with practices in southwestern Germany and Switzerland. With the help of hypnosis-supported psychotherapy, he primarily treats people with persistent psychological conditions. His practice focuses on anxiety disorders, pathological compulsions, and psychosomatic illnesses. His therapeutic offerings mainly include classical and modern hypnosis applications and the dreamland therapy he developed himself.

Copying, publishing, and sharing with third parties are only permitted with the written consent of the author. Please observe the notes on copyright and usage.

Distribution, publication, and copying in any form are prohibited and subject to damages.

Notes on Copyright and Usage

Copying, publishing, and sharing with third parties is prohibited and only permitted with the written consent of the author. Please observe the following copyright and usage guidelines.

This work has been carefully crafted and created to the best of the author's knowledge and personal experience. It comprises text templates and application guidelines for professional hypnosis sessions. The author is a licensed psychotherapist with extensive experience in psychotherapy, coaching, and personal training using hypnotic techniques and methods. Nevertheless, the author and the publisher assume no liability for the accuracy of information, instructions, and advice, nor for any typographical errors. The author and publisher accept no responsibility or liability for the application of these texts and recommendations with clients or patients, nor for any potential consequences or unexpected reactions. It is expressly noted that the application of therapeutic and advisory techniques and formulations lies solely and entirely within the responsibility of the practitioner. This also applies to adherence to the boundaries of legally regulated medical and therapeutic practices. The fact that a book containing action proposals is freely available for sale does not imply that its application with clients or patients is permitted for everyone.

Copying, publishing, and sharing with third parties are only permitted with the written consent of the author. Please observe the notes on copyright and usage.

Distribution, publication, and copying in any form are prohibited and subject to damages.

Copying, publishing, and sharing with third parties are only permitted with the written consent of the author. Please observe the notes on copyright and usage.

Distribution, publication, and copying in any form are prohibited and subject to damages.

Table of Contents

Introduction 9

Hypnosis 1 11

Hypnosis 2 16

Hypnosis 3 20

Hypnosis 4 26

Hypnosis 5 31

Hypnosis 6 36

Hypnosis 7 41

Hypnosis 8 46

Hypnosis 9 52

Hypnosis 10 57

Overview of All Titles in the Series "Ten Hypnoses" 61

Copying, publishing, and sharing with third parties are only permitted with the written consent of the author. Please observe the notes on copyright and usage.

Distribution, publication, and copying in any form are prohibited and subject to damages.

Copying, publishing, and sharing with third parties are only permitted with the written consent of the author. Please observe the notes on copyright and usage.

Distribution, publication, and copying in any form are prohibited and subject to damages.

Introduction

The series "Ten Hypnoses" is very well known in Germany, Austria, and Switzerland as a collection of texts for therapeutic work and is used by numerous psychotherapeutic practices, doctors, therapists, coaches, and other helping professionals. I am pleased to now be able to offer these texts in other countries as well.

Most therapists have their own methods for inducing and deepening trance as well as for exiting trance. Therefore, I have focused on the main part of the hypnosis. The texts in this book can be integrated as the main part into any hypnosis process. The texts in this collection use various hypnosis techniques. I will not explain these in detail, as I assume that users have the appropriate training. It is also not necessary to understand the exact structure or functioning of the different parts. The texts can simply be read aloud, and they will have their effect.

Decide for yourself which text best suits your client or patient at any given time. You can also combine passages

Copying, publishing, and sharing with third parties are only permitted with the written consent of the author. Please observe the notes on copyright and usage.

from different texts. It is not about using all ten hypnoses in sequence. It is a selection of possibilities.

I want to emphasize that books cannot replace therapy. Psychotherapy or other therapeutic treatments involve much more. A careful diagnosis is the necessary basis for deciding on the use of methods, including whether hypnosis or one of my texts should be used. Even in this case, preparatory discussions, follow-up discussions during the session, and of course, a therapeutic concept for the sequence of sessions and the content approaches are essential parts of therapy. This cannot and should not be achieved with a collection of texts.

In any case, I wish you much success in your work and I am pleased if my text templates can contribute in a small way.

Ingo Michael Simon

Hypnosis 1

Goal Setting and Willpower Strengthening

You have a goal ... ... You want to go out among people with joy again, to feel comfortable there ... ... For a long time, you withdrew, but now that's over ... ... Your decision is firm ... ... You want to go out again with ease and joy ... ... meet friends maybe or simply take a pleasant walk through the city ... ... with a sense of freedom and serenity in your thoughts ... ... with relaxation in your body ... ... and with the good feeling of doing something good for yourself ... ... Right now, you can focus on this goal very well ... ... very well ... ... and that's why now is the perfect time to start ... ... to start your new, free life ... ... right now the starting signal sounds ... ... right now ... ... So let's go ... ... let's take an important step today ... ... an important step into your new, free life ... ... very good ... ... You are doing very well to embrace this and really start now ... ...

Mental Alignment

Thoughts help us ... ... sometimes they even control us ... ... That can slow us down or help us ... ... and today your thoughts are only going to help you ... ... today your thoughts will help you be free and stay free ... ... So first, align your thoughts to change ... ... A very special thought that is now possible begins ... ... You speak a new truth in your mind ... ... You say ... ... I feel comfortable around other people because I can breathe freely ... ... a rather simple thought ... ... maybe you think it's too simple ... ... It's often the simple thoughts that can help us ... ... simple thoughts can slow us down or disturb us ... ... but a simple thought can also help a lot, can free you ... ... if it's the right thought at the right time ... ... I feel comfortable around other people because I can breathe freely ... ... if it's the right thought at the right time ... ... I feel comfortable around other people because I can breathe freely ... ... That is the right thought ... ... that is the fitting thought ... ... the thought of the coming days and weeks ... ...

Somatic Alignment (Body Suggestion)

Now concentrate on your body feeling ... ... especially feel your breathing ... ... and feel how your body expands with each breath ... ... Your body matches your thought ... ... breathe freely ... ... That's what you can do ... ... breathe freely ... ... That's what you do ... ... breathe freely ... ... breathe deeply in and feel your chest expand ... ... You can do it ... ... You can breathe freely, right now in this beautiful relaxation it works and outside it works just as well ... ... there too you can breathe freely and feel comfortable ... ... just like now ... ... exactly like now ... ... What is possible now is possible every day ... ... breathe freely and feel comfortable ... ... even in crowds, breathe freely and feel comfortable ... ...

Emotional Alignment (Feeling Suggestion)

Feel even deeper your actual feeling right now ... ... the feeling of deep relaxation and inner calm ... ... But you find even more beautiful feelings deep inside you ... ... feelings of serenity and freedom ... ... absence of fear ... ... now, at this moment, you cannot feel any fear at all ... ... not even if you wanted to ... ... You could remember fear, but you stay calm and serene ... ... very relaxed ... ... So it's possible to think about a crowd and still stay serene ... ... It's possible and you can do it ... ... You are doing it right now ... ... and this connection is new and right ... ... crowd and serenity ... ... that is new and right ... ... crowd and serenity ... ... and if you think you should be even more serene ... ... even calmer ... ... even more relaxed ... ... then enjoy the calm even more ... ... concentrate even more on the calm and let it become more intense ...

Behavioral Alignment

You can achieve even more ... ... You can go out again ... ... You have the power because today you learn how you can regain and keep the power over your feelings and your body ... ... so you are the one who can act ... ... so now you also prepare to be active ... ... to go out again ... ... maybe at first for a few minutes ... ... for a little walk in the fresh air ... ... in the middle of the city ... ... You decide when to go out ... ... You decide who has the power ... ... You decide for yourself ... ... for your power ...

Outlook and Vision

You can already imagine how wonderful it will be once you have fully succeeded in being free and serene among people again ... ... because you have succeeded in letting go of fear forever ... ... because you have succeeded in controlling your feelings ... ... because you have succeeded in prioritizing serenity and freedom ... ... You can enjoy life again because you are free ... ... You imagine it right now ... ... like a glimpse ahead ... ... a glimpse into the future ... ... But maybe it's not a glimpse into the future, but a glimpse into the present, because you have already become free ...

Summary

You have decided ... ... You go out again and it succeeds better than before ... ... it succeeds really well ... ... A right and good thought fills you ... ... the thought ... ... I feel comfortable around other people because I can breathe freely ... ... You can feel at any moment that breathing freely is possible ... ... Breathing in expands your chest and gives you the feeling of freedom ... ... Your feelings fully align with freedom and serenity ... ... and you take control ... ... You think ... ... I feel comfortable around other people because I can breathe freely ... ... Then you realize that you have the power ... ... only you have the power and you decide ... ... only you decide ... ... You decide that you are stronger than any fear could be ... ... You decide to go among people ... ... You ... ...

Distribution, publication, and copying in any form are prohibited and subject to damages.

Copying, publishing, and sharing with third parties are only permitted with the written consent of the author. Please observe the notes on copyright and usage.

Hypnosis 2

Goal Setting and Motivation

... ... You know it is right to initiate a big change now, to end the fear in crowds / at unfamiliar places as soon as possible ... ... Very good how you focus on this goal, the end of fear ... ...

... ... Therefore, you are ready to address everything associated with the fact that there has been fear among people / at unfamiliar places so far ... ... Very good how you go much deeper now and process the deep causes of fear ... ...

... ... Yes, you start now with the thorough and detailed processing of all entanglements of fear, because that frees you already today ... ... Very good how you do exactly that ... ...

Command to the Subconscious

... ... You know that your inner center can help you and that is why you have chosen trance to end the fear and finally be free … … Very good how you trust your inner center now … …

… … So now you allow your inner center to untangle and dissolve all entanglements and confusions in your deep emotions because then you regain self-confidence and self-assurance, and the fear dissolves completely … … Very good how you engage with your inner center and feel that exactly there all entanglements and confusions are truly being resolved … … and the fear disappears by itself … …

… … Yes, you now allow your inner center to untangle and dissolve all entanglements and confusions in depth and thus end the fear … … Very good how you do exactly that … …

Consciousness Steering

… … You know that you will reach your goal faster if you deal with yourself patiently and considerately and align your thoughts constructively … … Very good how you do that, to align and guide your thoughts patiently and considerately and constructively … …

… … So now you decide to think and feel patiently and considerately … … Yes, I trust my inner center and therefore myself … … Very good how you do that, truly trusting your inner center and feeling that it really resolves all fear and builds new self-confidence ... ...

... ... Yes, you now guide your thoughts patiently and considerately to trust your inner center and experience the dissolution of fear ... ... You now guide your thoughts patiently and considerately ... ... Very good how you do exactly that ... ...

Processing in the Subconscious

... ... Your inner center knows that there are uncertainties and memories that led to the fear among people ... ... Your inner center knows all the causes and connections, all the origins in your emotions that need to be resolved now ... ... Very good how your deep inner self manages to handle all this for you ... ... Your inner center gladly takes care of all this for you and processes the deep and old fear, and then it dissolves completely and forever ... ... Very good how quickly your inner center can handle this task ... ... Very good how you work together with your inner center ... ...

... ... Yes, your inner center is already taking care of resolving the fear right now, examining it and analyzing it, and can thus easily and securely process it ... ... thus the fear dissolves, and you feel self-assurance and lightness again ... ... Very good how you do that, now already feeling self-assurance and lightness ... ...

Outlook

... ... You know that deep in your emotions a special change has indeed occurred and continues to occur ... ... Very good how you do that, to engage in a real change ... ...

... ... Therefore, you are also sure that your inner center continues to help you because all your abilities and possibilities lie there ... ... Very good how you do that, always trusting your inner center in your waking everyday life ... ...

... ... Yes, you trust your inner center unconditionally ... ... for the end of fear and for self-confidence and self-assurance among people, even at unfamiliar places ... ... Very good how quickly the end of fear is possible ... ...

Hypnosis 3

Anchor Technique (Olfactory Anchor, Post-Hypnotic)

As an anchor (or trigger), a stimulus that evokes a specific feeling or thought is called. It is a signal perceived by the client that then initiates an internal process. The established anchor then replaces the suggestion. In everyday life, a client can use an anchor to initiate or create a desired state without a trance state. Numerous stimuli can be used as anchors/triggers. I work with the following possibilities, which I also use in the series "Ten Hypnoses": body anchors (closing the hand, pressing the thumb pad ...), visual anchors (symbols, word cards ...), acoustic anchors (signal sounds like mobile phone ringing, melodies ...), olfactory anchors (fragrance oils ...), haptic anchors (comfort stones, talismans ...). I also differentiate between peri-hypnotic and post-hypnotic anchors. Peri-hypnotic anchors are those primarily used during hypnosis by the therapist to establish the anchor and then trigger it repeatedly as a supplement to suggestions and visualizations. Post-hypnotic anchors are primarily set up for the time after the session so the client can help themselves with them.

Preparing the Anchor Technique

You have a goal ... ... You want to be able to move alone outside and feel comfortable ... ... You also want to be able to be in crowds and feel comfortable ... ... You know the difficult situation of going out alone ... ... standing on large squares or crossing them ... ... or being in a large crowd ... ... You know the feeling of fear ... ... Fear that something might happen, you could faint or have to vomit ... ... But you still remember how it used to be, because you used to be able to go out well ... ... could stand or cross a large square alone ... ... could be in dense crowds and be without fear ... ... today you return to that ... ... back to normality ... ... You need help, something that can help you directly to endure a difficult situation ... ... or better yet, not get into a difficult situation at all ... ... just be there and feel comfortable ... ... just be among people and feel comfortable ... ... That's possible ... ... It's even better than you think ... ... It's possible with the help of an anchor ... ... an anchor is a tool that helps you stay calm ... ... calm when you're outside, in the open ... ... calm, especially in crowds ... ... maybe you already have an idea of how it works with the anchor ... ... or you wonder how it works exactly and are curious ... ... There are many ways to set up an anchor ... ... You can use an olfactory anchor, which sounds very special and that's exactly what it is ... ... a very special anchor ... ... a scent anchor ... ... that means that a smell or better said a scent can help you ... ... Your anchor is a very special scent that I have here in a small bottle ... ... Maybe you're already wondering how it smells ... ... or you wonder if you already know this scent and today will only find out that it can be your calming scent ... ... or you are just curious to experience the calm ... ... to be able to create the calm yourself again and again with your calming scent ...

Creating the Desired Emotional State

Now you feel calm and relaxed ... ... that's good, very, very good ... ... because that's how it must be when you're outside ... ... that's how it must be when you're among people ... ... so calm it must be and remain ... ... Now feel the calm and let it become very clear ... ... perceive the calm ... ... and if you think it should become even calmer inside you, then just breathe deeply in and exhale slowly and long ... ... because then it automatically becomes calmer ... ... calmer all by itself ... ... and imagine you were outside, in the open ... ... all alone and as calm as now ... ... You can be calm now and imagine being outside ... ... Here and now it's very easy because it's a fantasy ... ... and every fantasy that corresponds to your desire makes you calm and stay calm ... ... and it corresponds to your desire to be able to be outside and calm ... ... Feel your serenity ... ... Feel your relaxation ... ... You can do it really well and you're doing it well ... ... Both are now present, the crowd and the relaxation, just like before ... ... Everything is good now ... ... Let both be there ... ... the idea of the crowd and your calm ...

Setting Up the Anchor

Now in the real relaxation and calm everything around you becomes unimportant ... ... Now it's only about this feeling of calm ... ... calm when imagining the crowd ... ... calm when imagining being alone outside ... ... and this calm now becomes very clear ... ... As it is now, it can be every day, even and especially outside and among people ... ... it works ... ... just like now ... ... every day just like now ... ... It's very simple ... ... You can enter this feeling every day and then feel comfortable ... ... It works again and again, even and especially when it gets difficult ... ... Then it suddenly becomes easy to feel calm again ... ... Then it suddenly becomes easy to be outside and stay outside ... ... Then it suddenly becomes easy to be among people and stay among people ... ...

... ... [Open the bottle with the aroma and move it towards the client's nose; hold it there] ... ...

... ... Now breathe deeply in and consciously perceive the smell you sense ... ... a pleasant smell ... ... at the same time you clearly feel that you are calm ... ... Your good feeling and this smell you perceive now merge together ... ... They belong together ... ... This smell and inner calm belong very closely together ... ... This smell means: Yes, I am and remain calm! ... ... Yes, I am and remain calm ... ... Very good ... ...

... ... [Now take the bottle away and close it] ... ...

Consolidation (Post-Hypnotic Command)

Continue to breathe calmly and enjoy the calm ... ... Now give yourself attention and trust your subconscious that supports you in always reaching this state quickly, simply by smelling the scent I just presented to you ... ... and whenever you feel the fear might return, you open the bottle and smell the scent of calm and relax immediately and stay calm ... ... Your calming scent lets you become calm always and everywhere ...

Hypnosis 4

Preparation and Willpower Strengthening

You have often felt uncomfortable when you went out, were alone ... ... You have also often felt uncomfortable in crowds ... ... maybe it is more appropriate to say that you were afraid, because you could clearly feel fear ... ... You want to end that, want to regain control over your life ... ... You want to control the fear and then let it go or banish it forever ... ... You are ready, more ready than ever before ... ... Everything has its time, and liberation also needs the right time ... ... That time is now ... ... Now is the right time ... ... Today you can conquer fear ... ... without struggle ... ... only with calm ...

Distancing Active Thoughts

Now all thoughts can go ... ... all thoughts can move on like clouds in the sky ... ... No one can hold the clouds ... ... not even the sky ... ... The wind drives all clouds away ... ... They simply drift away in the wind ... ... it cannot be otherwise ... ... and just like that your thoughts simply move on ... ... Thoughts come and go ... ... They pass by and it gradually becomes quieter inside you ... ... It's as if all thoughts are immediately blown away by the wind ... ... and nothing is important anymore ... ... only calm ... ... and it gradually becomes calmer and calmer inside you ... ... quieter and quieter inside you ... ... You sink into yourself ... ... immerse completely in your feeling ... ... in the feeling of calm ... ... calm inside you ... ... Maybe it is that your body feels lighter and lighter ... ... or you feel a very pleasant heaviness inside you ... ... maybe it's like that ... ... or like that ... ... but all thoughts move on ... ... It becomes calmer and quieter ... ... It's as if you look at the sky and see no more clouds because all are immediately dissolved in the wind ... ... and every cloud that might arise immediately dissolves in the wind ... ... The sky inside you becomes clear ... ... You can see everything clearly ... ... see everything very clearly ...

Presentation of the Affirmation

Then you see a cloud in the sky ... ... a large, white cloud ... ... But it also gradually dissolves ... ... and you see that behind the white cloud there is a thick, black writing in the sky ... ... Something is written in the sky for you ... ... in thick letters ... ... clearly, very clearly ... ... but first, the white cloud must completely dissolve in the wind so you can see the thick writing clearly ... ... very clearly ... ... The cloud dissolves ... ... The cloud and all thoughts dissolve ... ... all thoughts disappear in the wind ... ... dissolve and you can see the writing ... ... There, written in the sky, it says ... ...

I feel comfortable under the open sky and crowds are a safe environment.

... [Read the affirmation slowly and a little louder than the previous text, to highlight it a bit. Then pause for about 30 seconds before continuing to read.] ...

Influencing and Deepening the Affirmation

Let these words flow deep into your inner self ... ... accept them and let them work for you ... ... Allow yourself calm and serenity now ... ... calm and serenity ... ... and feel how you feel now ... ... feel the calm you now have ... ... that's all you need ... ... that's really all you need ... ... because now you have calm and a sky writing ... ... calm and clear words for you in the sky ... ... and both merge together ... ... it happens naturally ... ... happens deep inside you, without struggle and without effort ... ... it just happens, because this sentence becomes a belief ... ... an attitude in you ... ... a very deep attitude in your feeling ... ... a very deep attitude in your subconscious ... ... Everything is calm inside you ... ... You can feel the calm ... ... You feel the calm because it cannot be otherwise ... ... and everything changes in this moment ... ... everything changes inside you, because your sky writing becomes a stable attitude ... ... It sounds too simple to be true ... ... but it really is true ... ... and soon you can feel it ... ... you can feel it now because you feel good ... ... and in your waking everyday life you can soon feel it too, because even when you wake up, you feel good ... ... You feel good in your everyday life ... ... also outside you feel good ... ... also in groups of people you feel good ...

Repetition and Integration of the Affirmation

Deep inside you, the words work, which you can look at again in the sky and take in even deeper inside you ... ...

I feel comfortable under the open sky and crowds are a safe environment.

...... Now give yourself a moment where you don't have to think about anything ...... Just be there and enjoy the feeling of calm, that's enough ...... more than enough ...... Everything important is done ...

Consolidation (Post-Hypnotic Command)

It's time ...... You have internalized a new attitude that unfolds more every day ...... because deep inside you, these words are written that you heard today ...... the words of the sky ...... Your organism remembers this every day ...... and when you're outside, in the city or among people, a quick look at the sky is enough to remind yourself and your deep inner self of your deep attitude and immediately awaken the feeling of calm ...... with just one single look at the sky, you become calmer and freer ...... every day ...... just like today ...

Hypnosis 5

Goal Setting and Preparation

You have realized that it's time to overcome fear ... ... to be stronger than the fear ... ... to perceive it and then let it go ... ... You have the firm will to conquer fear and thus find yourself again ... ... because behind the fear there are many pleasant feelings and interests that you couldn't perceive so well in the fear of the past ... ... That should now change ... ... You can and will recognize and feel all the beautiful feelings behind the fear again ... ... You can and will free yourself from the fear ... ... and replace the freed-up space with curiosity and openness ... ... joy in meeting other people ... ... You can do it ... ... you succeed excellently ... ... Today you take the decisive step ... ... Now you set off ... ... now ... ...

Perspective Change

You have often experienced the fear as inexplicable, couldn't comprehend it yourself ... ... You then perhaps thought that you were afraid of people ... ... afraid of other people or of the crowd of people around you when you are out ... ... in the city or on a market place ... ... You think about it now ... ... Now, in the calm of deep relaxation, you can think about fear without really feeling it ... ... You can remember it, look at it like a headline, but you stay calm ... ... In fact, this means that you have already left a large part of the fear behind you ... ... that you can also calmly experience situations that used to scare you a lot ... ... in imagination it works and what works in imagination is fundamentally also possible in the waking everyday life ... ... Look around your inner market place, imagine a situation where you were once afraid and call this place your inner market place ... ... There you were afraid and thought you were afraid of people ... ... but on closer inspection, that's not true because you didn't fear they would harm you ... ... That's not how it was with you ... ... So you weren't afraid of the crowd, but afraid in the crowd ... ... That's a difference ... ... an important difference ... ... it's like having a cold or stomachache that you could have had in the market ... ... The market and the crowd wouldn't have been the cause, but the place of occurrence ... ... Deep inside you, this perspective on fear helps you ... ... to know that not the crowd is the reason for the fear, but only the place of the fear ... ... It comes from deep inside you, originated there in a time of threat or in a time when you needed help and didn't get it ... ... maybe even without having felt your inner distress at that time ... ... that's possible too ... ...

Re-Evaluation of Own Experiences

Now remember a situation of fear ... ... fear in a crowd ... ... and maybe it wasn't even that many people who were there ... ... maybe everything was too close and too tight and you didn't know what to do ... ... The fear only came in contact with people, always when avoiding or running away wasn't so well possible ... ... because you thought something terrible could happen, you could faint or have to vomit and then be exposed to looks ... ... Today you can imagine that it would have been easier for you if the judgment of others wasn't so important to you, if you could have focused entirely on overcoming the fear ... ... then you might have found helpers in the crowd ... ... then people around you could even have been a signal for a little more safety ... ... You wouldn't have been alone with your fear ... ... Imagine there was someone who would have helped you ... ... someone who would have told you that it wasn't your fault that you were afraid ... ... Someone who would have helped you out of there ... ... or even several ... ... then the crowd would have suddenly turned into a safety zone ... ... but that wasn't so easy in the past ... ... and possibly there was no one who really wanted or could help ... ... but today you imagine that the fear wasn't there because of the crowd, but despite the many people there ... ... They only suddenly seemed so threatening, but they weren't ... ... The fear was the threat ... ... but today you can control the fear ...

Action Change

In your fantasy, in your imagination, you stand in a crowd and remain calm ... ... You move very calmly and naturally and go your way on this inner market ... ... Then you stand in the middle of the market place and shout as loud as you can ... ... You are not my fear ... ... You are not my fear ... ... and you feel calm and relaxed ... ... You have the feeling that the fear is moving away from you ... ... Then you say loudly and clearly ... ... I am here, and I am strong ... ... I am here, and I am strong ... ... and again your fear moves further away from you ... ... and you see the friendly faces of the people ... ... feel their recognition and serenity ... ... You see the many people in your imagination and feel free because you don't need to explain or hide your fear ... ... It was a part of you and maybe still is in a special way ... ... as a memory ... ... as an experience ... ... but in the crowd, you are free ... ... completely free and serene ...

Consolidation

You now feel the inner calm and relaxation ... ... You know that you can control the fear yourself ... ... that you can let go of the fear because you know it is a part of you that you can control ... ... today in your imagination and also in your everyday life when you are awake ... ... People have nothing to do with it ... ... they are just there ...

Hypnosis 6

Goal Setting and Preparation

You want to overcome fear ... ... fear in the open ... ... because somehow it has happened that you feel uncomfortable outside ... ... outside and also where there are many people ... ... You don't know why it has happened ... ... You haven't done anything wrong ... ... no one can say why it is so ... ... sometimes everything is too much, the burdens of life are too great, and then strange feelings arise ... ... You could get a stomach ulcer or an incomprehensible fear ... ... But it's not important to understand where it comes from or why it's there ... ... it's important to know how you can get out of it ... ... Because above all, you want to experience the end of this fear ... ... There should be a helper who can quickly help you out of a fear situation ... ... one you can always have near you ... ... there is one ... ... There is this helper in you ...

Creating a Place of Encounter

You can meet your inner helper, can encounter them ... ... Your inner helper is not a ritual and not a therapist's trick ... ... They are simply a part of you ... ... We all have different parts or aspects within us ... ... strong and weak ones ... ... angry and serene ones ... ... cautious and clumsy ones ... ... At home, you feel safe, there you feel your strong part ... ... outside you feel the fearful part ... ... and deep inside you, there is a place where you can meet all parts ... ... can meet yourself ... ... deep in your feeling ... ... deep in your imagination ... ... You let yourself fall into your own feeling and find a place within you, a quiet place ... ... a completely empty room where you feel comfortable because you are within yourself ... ... are close to yourself ... ... to all your strengths ... ... You are at a place of inner encounter ... ... You encounter yourself ... ... stand facing yourself ... ... a special part of your personality ...

Encountering the Inner Helper

Deep inside you, you stand facing yourself ... ... a special part of you ... ... This person inside you looks like you ... ... and introduces themselves as your inner helper ... [Please adjust to the client's gender] ... and maybe you wonder how a part of yourself can actually help you ... ... wonder how exactly that can work ... ... If you are your own inner helper, then isn't your fear your helper too? ... ... Maybe it's exactly like that ... ... maybe even the fear can help you ... ... if it comes to the right place ... ... to the place of remembrance, because that's where it belongs ... ... to the place of remembrance ...

Confrontation and Clarification

You think about how difficult and burdensome the time of fear has been and how much you wish it could end now ... ... Then you ask the person inside you what you can do to overcome the fear ... ... then you ask yourself what you can do to overcome the fear ... ... and your helper holds a book in their hands ... ... They tell you that it is possible to overcome the fear ... ... inside you, it has already happened because there is strength and courage ... ... sufficient strength and courage ... ... and this helper tells you that they have overcome the fear ... ... You learn that this likeness of you that you have met here is the bearer of your fear ... ... but exactly this part, which had the fear, has also overcome it ... ... You ask how that was achieved and learn that your inner helper has fully accepted the fear, accepted that it belongs to you ... ... Your helper opens the book ... ... it is blank, it is unwritten ... ... and you get a pen to write in the book ... ... You write in it ... ... The fear was a part of me ... ... The fear was a part of me ... ... Then your helper closes the book of fear ...

... ... Deep inside you, there is the place of remembrance ... ... where all life experiences eventually arrive ... ... as a memory that remains ... ... but is handed over to the past ... ... and that's exactly where your helper takes the book of fear ... ... That's exactly where you yourself take the book of fear ... ... to the place of remembrance ... ... and at the same time, you feel the feeling of freedom more clearly inside you ... ... Still, you stand in this special place inside you, which becomes a symbol for every place outside ... ... in the inner vastness, you can feel comfortable ... ... and outside, on squares and among people, you can feel just as comfortable, because there too your inner helper immediately brings the book of fear to the place of remembrance ... ... because fear belongs to the past ... ... You don't need it anymore ... ... The fearful part in you takes the fear to the place of remembrance ... ... because precisely this fearful part can be a helper to you ... ... precisely the fearful part is the one that moves to help you ... ... Today in your imagination and in your waking everyday life from now on, when you go out and are among people ... ... just as today your fearful part takes the book of fear away ...

Consolidation (Post-Hypnotic Command)

It is like an inner ritual that runs by itself ... ... As soon as you go out, the fearful part in you writes the fear in the book and takes the book of fear to the place of remembrance, far away from you ... ... so fear cannot even arise ... ... so the active part of you that goes out and meets people remains calm and serene ... ... calm and serene ... ... Your fearful part remains your helper inside ... ... because precisely this part of you takes the fear away, so you, the active one, remain strong and capable of action ... ... You are and remain strong and capable of action ... ... strong and capable of action ... ... now and always, when you go out ... ... now and always, when you are among people ...

Hypnosis 7

Goal Setting and Preparation

You want to change everything today ... ... Your decision is firm ... ... You want to control the fear ... ... You have experienced it differently, but today you take the helm ... ... Your decision is good because this way you regain your life ... ... can move freely again and go where you want ... ... because exactly that is your goal ... ... to be able to move freely again ... ... go out and be among people and feel comfortable ... ... You won't let yourself be stopped ... ... You won't let the fear slow you down or hinder you ... ... You go against the fear ... ... today you go against the fear ... ... and find the strength in you because there is enough strength in you to reach your goal ... ... There is enough courage in you to reach your goal ... ... Today the change begins ... ... and it is remarkable how strong you are in this and how persistent you can be ... ... more persistent than the fear, because you are really stronger ...

Somato-Emotional Change

Body and feeling are closely connected ... ... Fear shows itself in a timid body posture and courage and strength show themselves in an upright, strong posture ... ... Self-confidence shows itself in a strong posture ... ... and our body adapts to our feelings ... ... Your body adapts to your feelings ... ... and your thoughts, because strong thoughts also bring your body into an upright and stable position and fear has to give way ... ... Today you adjust more than ever to this thought of your own strength ... ... to the thought that you can really be strong ... ... and your body helps you with that ... ... You adjust to the thought that you are really strong and your body helps you with that ... ... It's truly remarkable how quickly your body posture already changes, even in calm ... ... quite remarkable how your body is already adjusting to your new courage and inner leadership ... ... Your body prepares everything for you so that you can walk upright and with your head held high through any crowd and feel good ... ... It is indeed possible because you want it that way ... ... because you now, in the trance, want it that way ... ... because your body follows your thoughts and your feelings follow your body ... ... First there is the thought of strength and self-assurance ... ... then follows the body posture of strength and self-assurance ... ... right now ... ... and then follows the feeling of strength and self-assurance ... ... right now ... ... You now let an inner image arise of how good it feels when you walk through a crowd confidently and strong and feel completely safe ... ... This day has now come because today you are already adjusting to it as intensively as possible ... ... You become stronger ... ... Your body takes an ever more stable posture ... ... If you feel deeply into your body and become aware of it, you can clearly feel how it changes ... ... right now in this moment ... ... Your breath becomes wider ... ... much wider ... ... Your chest feels the opening and freedom of deep inhalation ... ... You feel it because your body feels bigger ... ... bigger and stronger ... ... Quite remarkable how clearly your body already signals your new strength ...

And you can perceive it now ... ... You can clearly perceive it ... ... your strength ... ... your inner strength ... ... So all your thoughts also align with being strong and walking through the crowd as a matter of course ... ... It's so everyday in your imagination that you can actually do it ... ... much better and much faster than you thought ... ... Today you can feel it ... ... You have the power and strength ... ... You have the power ... ... You feel the determination ... ... It is now time to let go of any fear ... ... You make it clear to yourself that your fear is only a memory ... ... a memory of a past time ... ... Every day begins anew and every day you can begin anew ... ... with your new power and strength ... ... Isn't it quite excellent that you can even feel comfortable in the crowd? ... ... You have gone so far inwardly that you can now free yourself from old thought patterns and habits that you no longer need ... ... You are strong and tall ... ... and just as strong and tall you go out into the city ... ... among people to feel even more comfortable, because today a new part of your life begins ... ... a chapter full of courage and sovereignty ... ... a time that lets you become stronger and stronger ... ... And your body still shows you how strong you have become ... ... Pay attention to your body feeling once more and feel this deep strength ... ... this constructive tension ... ... this posture that shows ... ... Yes! I am strong ... ... Yes! I face my fear ... ... Yes! I conquer the uncertainty and become stronger ... ... just like in this moment ... ... You can now fully enjoy this new and good feeling ... ... make this vision of a free and strong future very intense and thus turn your inner vision into an outer reality ... ... because everything you think can become reality ... ... Already today you experience your new reality ... ... courage and strength ... ... calm and sovereignty ...

... ... Now feel deeply into your body ... ... perceive the feeling of your body ... ... relaxed and with posture ... ... your body helps you because whenever you think you need more courage and strength, you can focus on your body and feel exactly this feeling ... ... strength in your body ... ... relaxation and at the same time powerful posture ...

Consolidation (Post-Hypnotic Command)

Every day you can remind your body to help you ... ... to help you be strong and stay strong ... ... You simply stand in front of a mirror and imagine that you have the power ... ... and then you can observe that your body takes on a strong and proud posture ... ... that your body takes posture ... ... and you immediately feel that it makes you even stronger ... ... You feel your strength in your body and feel how you feel even stronger ... ... just like now ... ... exactly like now ...

Hypnosis 8

Ideomotorics refers to the phenomenon that our body follows our feelings and thoughts with movements. In everyday life, this following shows itself as body posture, muscle tension, and movement patterns of a person that naturally change with the mood and thoughts. In trance, ideomotoric signals can be used to receive information that the client cannot actively communicate. For example, the subconscious can answer questions with an agreed finger signal. Naturally, ideomotoric reactions can also be used suggestively, such as in arm levitations and catalepsies. An ideomotoric approach strengthens trust in hypnosis and in one's ability to change, thereby promoting therapy.

Goal Setting and Preparation

You want to let go of the fear ... ... the fear in crowds and outside alone you want to let go and replace it with your own strength ... ... You want to take control again and possess and hold the power over your life ... ... You want to be self-determined and strong again ... ... want to move among people and feel calm and safe ... ... calm and safe ... ... That's why you are here today ... ... You are here to achieve exactly that ... ... and it can succeed for you today ... ... For this, I invite your subconscious to work with me and with you ... ... Your subconscious can help you and even more ... ... It can show you that it has replaced the fear with strength as soon as it is ready ... ... and maybe you wonder how quickly that can happen ... ... You will experience it in a few moments ... ...

Arm Levitation with Ideomotoric Command

Imagine your subconscious could make your arm light for you ... ... so light that your arm rises into the air as if weightless ... ... If your subconscious can do that, then it can also drive away the fear or make it light and build up strength for you ... ... Therefore, I agree with your subconscious on the following: Letting go of the fear should be shown by lightness ... ... and your new strength should be shown by rigidity and stability ... ... good ... ... That is done, because your body has understood me ... ... Now imagine there is a balloon tied to your arm ... ... filled with gas ... ... a balloon that rises upwards and pulls very hard on your arm and at the same time pulls the fear out of you ... ... The gas balloon rises up and pulls on your arm ... ... it pulls and pulls and pulls upwards and pulls your arm weightlessly into the air ... ... a huge gas balloon that becomes bigger and lighter and pulls your arm upwards with it ... ... You feel it, you can feel the pulling ... ... Let your arm simply rise up ... ... The huge balloon does the work for you ... ... You don't have to exert yourself ... ... You don't have to do anything, your subconscious does it for you ... ... The huge balloon rises into the sky ... ... flies into the sky and takes your arm with it ... ... your arm rises higher and higher ... ... higher and higher ... ... as if by itself your arm moves into the air, carried by the balloon ... ... your arm becomes lighter and lighter ... ... ever lighter ... ... feather-light becomes your arm and the balloon pulls it upwards ... ... Higher and higher rises the balloon ... ... yes, exactly like that ... ... higher and higher ... ... and your arm rises with it ... ... and it is very light ... ... goes as if by itself ... ... your arm becomes lighter and lighter and rises now ever higher ... ... Your arm rises higher and higher and your fear becomes light and dissolves ... ... Your fear becomes lighter and lighter and dissolves while your arm rises higher and higher ... ...

[Please stay with it. The suggestive connection between the rising arm and letting go of fear is already established. The continuous suggestion for the arm to rise will lead to the arm eventually rising, which has the effect of reducing fear. Repeat lightness and balloon suggestions until the arm moves – It will happen!]

… … Very good … … excellent … … your arm floats feather-light and the balloon continues to pull and hold your arm in this position … … your arm is held in this position and it is feather-light … … Your arm remains in this position and is light … … your fear is dissolved … … your fear is now dissolved and your arm remains light … … Simply open your eyes briefly, even then your arm remains in this position … … Open your eyes and look at your arm, it remains held in exactly this position …

[Always have clients look briefly at the levitating arm during arm levitations, otherwise it could be mistaken for an illusion. It is important for the levitating arm to be consciously experienced as it strengthens belief and trust in the possibilities of hypnosis. Don't worry – The arm will stay held. Complicated fractionations are not necessary.]

Catalepsy with Stabilization of the New

Now close your eyes again and continue to enjoy the calm ... ... Your arm remains in this position and now becomes very firm ... ... Your arm becomes very firm, completely immovable ... ... like iron, your arm becomes stiff and nothing and no one can move it anymore ... ... Your arm is held and becomes completely immovable ... ... stiff as iron ... ... stiff as iron, your arm is completely immovable ... ... I'll show you that your arm remains completely stiff ...

[Press against the arm, which will offer noticeable resistance. The client experiences that their arm is truly cataleptic. But don't overdo it, please! Gentle pressure! The connection between catalepsy and new strength has already been suggestively established. The cataleptic arm "proves" the inner change to the client.]

Releasing the Catalepsy and Ideomotorics

You have already achieved a lot ... ... your body has shown you what is possible ... ... The lightness of your arm shows you that fear has indeed been released because only under this condition could your arm follow the image of the gas balloon ... ... and the stiffness of your arm now shows you that new courage has arisen, that you have truly become stronger because only under this condition could your arm become stiff ... ... that was agreed with your subconscious and your subconscious never lies ... ... But now it is time for your subconscious to hand over the power to you ... ... and therefore the balloon disappears now, you don't need it anymore ... ... your arm becomes gradually heavier and sinks down again ... ... Your subconscious shows you again with this ... ... it shows you that you have the power ... ... that you really have the power to always let go of the fear and be strong ... ... only under this condition does your arm become movable and heavy ... ... and it does ... ... movable and heavy ... ... your arm becomes completely movable and sinks down ... ... [Stay with it! It will happen, even if the client is still skeptical. The heaviness suggestion prevails!] ... ...

Hypnosis 9

Preparation

You have a goal, an unshakeable and significant goal ... ... You want to let go of the fear ... ... You want to overcome the fear in crowds and make it disappear once and for all ... ... For this, hypnosis can be used, that's why you are here ... ... and today it should be a very special kind of hypnosis ... ... a hypnosis that works exactly like fear, only the other way around ... ... Maybe you wonder how that can work ... ... or you wonder how the fear actually works ... ... But in fact, you know it, because you know fear well ... ... It comes suddenly, is simply there ... ... You might have been in a shopping center or in a hall with many people and suddenly it was there ... ... then you did and tried many things, but it remained ... ... Imagine we do it the same way with the feeling of serenity and inner balance ... ... Exactly that is possible ... ... So let's do it ... ...

Pre-Assumption

You have often tried to fight the fear, sometimes even when it wasn't there yet ... ... and in fear you then tried to flee, from the people and somehow run away from the fear ... ... Today we do it differently ... ... The memory of fear can be there, also an idea of fear, that doesn't matter ... ... Then we add a vision of your goal, a very concrete vision, which I formulate as a goal for you in a short sentence ... ... and then we occupy ourselves with something completely different ... ... then we let the goal simply be there, just like the fear was there ... ... and your deep inner self, your subconscious has a lot of time and opportunity to let go of the fear and your inner self takes the opportunity to build serenity and balance for you ... ... for this, we need a thought that doesn't deal with fear and not with serenity ... ... How does that work? ... ... Well, a simple image that you imagine very intensely is enough ... ... the image of a full moon ... ... So simple? ... ... Yes, exactly ... ... so simple ... ... because the more you manage to concentrate on the image of the full moon and imagine it, the faster serenity and balance build up ... ... Fear could spread because you had nothing to counter it with ... ... that didn't work because it was so strong ... ... Today it's easier ... ... We occupy ourselves with your goal and then we counter nothing, make the way free for your goal ...

Current State and Goal Setting

And now concentrate on your goal ... ... You have experienced fear in groups of people ... ... That was the past ... ... Now it should be like this ... ...

Calm and balance inside and outside. Serenity in crowds

... [Place your palm on the client's solar plexus when stating the goal and then move it away. It's not necessary but helps a lot, because the goal is thus "anchored." Of course, you can also incorporate energetic techniques into the hypnosis. Make sure not to repeat the goal.] ...

Building the Emotionally Balancing Frame

Imagine you see a full moon above you ... ... a white full moon against a deep black background ... ... Everything is dark and black, and the moon shines round and bright ... ... Look at the moon and concentrate entirely on this image ...

… and slowly the moon becomes bigger … … it expands … … the moon becomes bigger and shines brighter … … with every breath it becomes bigger and bigger … … The full moon becomes a huge white ball in the night sky … … and with every breath it becomes bigger … … [Always on the client's inhalation] … … and bigger … … ever bigger becomes the moon … … it becomes bigger … … and bigger … …

… … and over time the white moon outshines the entire black night sky, which becomes completely white … … then it is so that the moon comes closer and closer to you … … like a huge, white light ball … … because it becomes bigger and bigger … … so big that it will soon touch the earth … … Imagine this image, recognize that this full moon consists of pure light … … Light that captures your body and soon surrounds it completely

… … and eventually the entire earth ball is enveloped by the white moonlight … … You immerse yourself completely in this white light and feel good … … and then the moonlight can become smaller again … … with every breath you let the moon become smaller again … … always with exhalation the moon becomes a little smaller and you can see the night sky again ... ... with every breath the moon becomes smaller ... ... until it finally stands as a full moon in the sky again ... ... and you feel good about it ... ... You feel really good ... ...

Dissolving the Energetic Frame

Now let your thoughts wander back and forth ... ... No thought is important now ... ... There is nothing more to do, because everything is already done ... ... everything is already finished ... ... maybe you felt that deep inside you a special change has happened ... ... or you just feel calm and balance inside you ... ... That was your goal ... ... and that's exactly how it should be when you go out again and meet people ... ...

Hypnosis 10

Arriving in the Land of Dreams

Make yourself comfortable, close your eyes … … and perceive the sounds of your surroundings … … You can hear the music in the room and let your imagination run wild … … imagine going to a beautiful place … … to a place of calm and contemplation … … to a place of quiet and reflection … … to a beautiful place deep inside you … … You also hear the sounds of everyday life … … because both are always there … … imagination and everyday life … … it only depends on the perspective … … if you concentrate on everyday life, you can hear the sounds of your surroundings clearly … … if you concentrate on your imagination and look deep inside yourself, then all that you can imagine and envision becomes much more present than everyday life … … then imagination and vision become the most important thing at this moment and everything becomes quieter … … With this vision of quiet and imagination, you go into the land of dreams, the most beautiful land that can be …

Confrontation, Clarification, and Creative Realignment

You stand in a huge garden and look around ... ... Many different plants grow here ... ... many are blooming right now, others even bear ripe fruit ... ... and again others are dried up and withered ... ... You think to yourself that this garden is like life itself ... ... many things bloom for a certain time and then pass away again ... ... others pass away before they could really bloom ... ... and everything has its time ... ... the fear also had its time, but this time should now be over because you are in the land of dreams to overcome the fear in crowds ... ... So you set off ... ... You follow a path that leads through this garden, and you find in the middle of this path a light blue ball, as big as a thick ball ... ... It is your wish ball ... ... You take it with you, tuck it under your arm, and wander through the garden ... ... The wish ball is very light, you can carry it quite easily ... ... Then you come to a beautiful bed with lots of blooming flowers ... ... and in this bed lies a golden ball ... ... You go closer and look into the golden ball ... ... and with a look into the ball, you remember a special success in your life, because this is the golden ball of your successes ... ... maybe you think you haven't had any special successes, but look closely ... ...

maybe you were once particularly proud of an achievement that may have seemed small but was very important to you ... ... a three-minus in mathematics or you ran faster than you thought ... ... Sometimes a three-minus feels like a one ... ... or you remember something that spontaneously comes to mind ... ... a small or even a very big success ... ... but there were successes in your life, and they are in this golden success ball ... ... You reach through the wall into the ball because in the land of dreams there are no limits for you ... ... You simply reach into this golden ball to grasp your own success power ... ... You grab your success power by sticking your hand into the golden ball and then closing it ... ... and then you place your success power into your light blue wish ball ... ... You stick your hand into the light blue wish ball and open it ... ... and your potential, all your possibilities, to experience success again, flow into your wish ball ... ... You go on and carry the ball of your wish fulfillment with you and inside it your own power ... ... success and overcoming ... ... success and overcoming ... ... your success ... ... and your overcoming of fear ...

Mindfulness and Self-Loyalty

You go on and reach the end of the garden ... ... Then you go to a beautiful flower meadow that adjoins the garden ... ... and you walk under a shining rainbow ... ... Everything seems so pure and clear ... ... and you find a nice place where you make yourself comfortable ... ... You lie down on the meadow and beside you lies the light blue wish ball that makes your dreams come true ... ... You rest and slowly fall asleep ... ... You dream a beautiful dream of going out again and meeting people ... ... even among many people you can be ... ... feel comfortable, surrounded by so many people ... ... with your wish ball under your arm, you walk in your freedom dream through a huge crowd and feel free ... ... free through your own power ... ... Here in the land of dreams it is possible, but the land of dreams is always there ... ... It lies deep inside you ... ... it has always been there ... ... I'm just telling you about it ... ...

Distribution, publication, and copying in any form are prohibited and subject to damages.

Overview of All Titles in the Series "Ten Hypnoses"

Volume 1: Smoking Cessation
Volume 2: Anxiety and Restlessness
Volume 3: Burnout
Volume 4: Reducing Overweight
Volume 5: Coping with the Past
Volume 6: Suicidal Thoughts and Attempts
Volume 7: Psycho-Oncology
Volume 8: Obsessions and Tics
Volume 9: Self-Confidence and Decision-Making
Volume 10: Grief Work
Volume 11: Psychosomatics
Volume 12: Chronic Pain
Volume 13: Depressive Thoughts
Volume 14: Panic Attacks
Volume 15: Domestic Violence, Victim Support
Volume 16: Post-Traumatic Stress
Volume 17: Exam Anxiety and Stage Fright
Volume 18: Anti-Violence Training, Offender Support
Volume 19: Addiction Tendencies
Volume 20: Social Phobia and Fear of Contact
Volume 21: Nail Biting
Volume 22: Self-Awareness and Self-Love
Volume 23: Teeth Grinding and Night Clenching
Volume 24: Feelings of Guilt
Volume 25: Fear in Crowds
Volume 26: Fear of Flying, Aviophobia
Volume 27: Fear in Enclosed Spaces, Claustrophobia
Volume 28: Tinnitus, Ear Noises
Volume 29: Fear of Heights
Volume 30: Neurodermatitis

Copying, publishing, and sharing with third parties are only permitted with the written consent of the author. Please observe the notes on copyright and usage.

Volume 31: Finding Inner Balance
Volume 32: Overcoming Loneliness
Volume 33: Fear of Illness, Hypochondria
Volume 34: Anticipatory Anxiety, Fear of Fear
Volume 35: Jealousy in Relationships
Volume 36: Driving Anxiety
Volume 37: New Start after Separation
Volume 38: Fear of Injections
Volume 39: Heart Anxiety Neurosis
Volume 40: Overcoming Resentment and Anger
Volume 41: Resolving Blockages and Positive Thinking
Volume 42: Stress Reduction, Stress Management
Volume 43: Body Relaxation
Volume 44: Deep Relaxation
Volume 45: Fear of the Dark
Volume 46: Falling Asleep and Staying Asleep
Volume 47: Compulsive Buying
Volume 48: Restless Legs Syndrome
Volume 49: Bulimia
Volume 50: Anorexia
Volume 51: Overcoming Nightmares
Volume 52: Imagined Deformity
Volume 53: Overcoming Distrust, Finding Trust
Volume 54: Processing Failures
Volume 55: Humiliation, Emotional Hurt
Volume 56: Distressing Compassion, Vicarious Suffering
Volume 57: Self-Forgiveness
Volume 58: Self-Awareness, Self-Confidence
Volume 59: Saying No
Volume 60: Assertiveness
Volume 61: Setting Boundaries and Self-Assertion
Volume 62: Decision-Making Ability

Volume 63: Success Orientation
Volume 64: Ruminating, Circular Thinking
Volume 65: Accepting Pregnancy
Volume 66: Birth Preparation
Volume 67: Spiritual Opening
Volume 68: Joy of Life and Inner Lightness
Volume 69: Patience and Inner Peace
Volume 70: Fibromyalgia and Rheumatism
Volume 71: Irritable Bowel Syndrome, Crohn's Disease
Volume 72: Fear of Nausea, Emetophobia
Volume 73: Stuttering and Cluttering, Speech Flow Disorders
Volume 74: Concentration and Knowledge Anchoring
Volume 75: Vitality and Spontaneity
Volume 76: Searching for Meaning and Finding Goals
Volume 77: Life Crises, Life Events
Volume 78: Workaholism, Goal Obsession
Volume 79: Helper Syndrome, Helpless Helpers
Volume 80: Medication Abuse
Volume 81: Gambling Addiction
Volume 82: Internet Addiction, Smartphone Addiction
Volume 83: Hoarding Disorder, Compulsive Collecting
Volume 84: Conspiracy Thoughts, Overvalued Ideas
Volume 85: Fear of Operations and Treatments
Volume 86: Fear of Aging
Volume 87: Travel Anxiety
Volume 88: Anxiety When Urinating, Paruresis
Volume 89: Fear of Intimacy and Togetherness
Volume 90: Fear of Blushing
Volume 91: Coming Out in Homosexuality
Volume 92: Charisma Training
Volume 93: Migraines and Chronic Headaches
Volume 94: Overcoming Allergies, Bronchial Asthma

Volume 95: Normalizing Blood Pressure
Volume 96: Compulsive Perfectionism
Volume 97: Sports Hypnosis, Motivation
Volume 98: Sports Hypnosis, Performance Enhancement
Volume 99: Determination and Focus
Volume 100: Encountering the Inner Child
Volume 101: Cravings, Binge Eating
Volume 102: Stimulating Metabolism
Volume 103: Bipolar Mood Swings
Volume 104: Borderline, Identity Crises
Volume 105: Hypomania, Euphoria, Mania
Volume 106: Restlessness, Agitation
Volume 107: Nervous Breakdown
Volume 108: Adjustment Disorders
Volume 109: Self-Alienation, Depersonalization
Volume 110: Ending Self-Pity
Volume 111: Primary Gain of Illness
Volume 112: Secondary Gain of Illness
Volume 113: Bullying, Victim Support
Volume 114: Letting Go of Envy and Jealousy
Volume 115: Fear of Spiders, Arachnophobia
Volume 116: Fear of Dogs or Cats
Volume 117: Fear of Strangers, Xenophobia
Volume 118: Excessive Worries, Generalized Anxiety
Volume 119: Strengthening Sense of Responsibility
Volume 120: Unrequited Love, Heartache
Volume 121: Work-Life Balance
Volume 122: Letting Go of Unattainable Goals
Volume 123: Allowing and Accepting Help
Volume 124: Letting Go of Adult Children
Volume 125: Tourette Syndrome
Volume 126: Life Changes and New Starts

Volume 127: Accepting Life in a Wheelchair
Volume 128: Understanding and Overcoming Homesickness
Volume 129: Understanding and Overcoming Wanderlust
Volume 130: Dizziness, Meniere's Disease
Volume 131: Overcoming Aggression
Volume 132: Cutting and Self-Harm
Volume 133: Hair Pulling, Trichotillomania
Volume 134: Postpartum Depression
Volume 135: For Relatives of Dementia Patients
Volume 136: Self-Harm, Artificial Disorders
Volume 137: Activating Self-Healing Powers
Volume 138: Preventing Depression Relapse
Volume 139: Reactive Psychoses, Follow-Up
Volume 140: Obsessive Thoughts and Impulses
Volume 141: Compulsive Checking
Volume 142: Compulsive Counting, Symmetry Obsession
Volume 143: Compulsive Washing, Cleanliness Obsession
Volume 144: Compulsive Questioning
Volume 145: Dissociative Paralysis
Volume 146: Phantom Pain
Volume 147: Overcoming Complaining
Volume 148: Hay Fever, Pollen Allergy
Volume 149: Sexual Abuse, Victim Support
Volume 150: Standing Strong Against Sexism, #metoo
Volume 151: Binge Eating
Volume 152: Overcoming Thoughts of Revenge
Volume 153: Detachment from the Aggressor, Stockholm Syndrome
Volume 154: Courage to Separate
Volume 155: Chronic Fatigue, Exhaustion
Volume 156: Fear of the Future, Existential Anxiety
Volume 157: Excessive Worry About Children
Volume 158: Fear of Failure

Volume 159: Ending Distrust and Control
Volume 160: Dejection, Dysphoria
Volume 161: Boreout, Chronic Boredom
Volume 162: Bipolar Disorders, Relapse Prevention
Volume 163: Mania, Relapse Prevention
Volume 164: Nihilism, Feelings of Worthlessness
Volume 165: Thumb Sucking
Volume 166: Being Brave
Volume 167: Being Proud
Volume 168: Overcoming Shyness
Volume 169: Being Able to Delegate Responsibility
Volume 170: Being Able to Show Emotions
Volume 171: Letting Go of Guilt, Victim Support
Volume 172: Processing Guilt, Offender Support
Volume 173: Mood Swings, Cyclothymia
Volume 174: Lack of Drive, Vital Sadness
Volume 175: Hearing Voices with Reality Reference
Volume 176: Confident Communication
Volume 177: Standing Up for Oneself
Volume 178: Taking New Paths
Volume 179: Confident Job Application
Volume 180: No Longer Being Taken Advantage Of
Volume 181: End of Submissiveness
Volume 182: Depressive Numbness
Volume 183: Mood Drops, Affective Incontinence
Volume 184: Mood Instability
Volume 185: Somatoform Disorders
Volume 186: Stomach Ulcer, Psychosomatic
Volume 187: Accepting Amputation
Volume 188: Overcoming and Letting Go of Hatred
Volume 189: Ending Accusations
Volume 190: Allowing Tears, Being Able to Cry

Volume 191: Finding and Sorting Repressed Feelings
Volume 192: Somatoform Pain
Volume 193: Living Autonomously
Volume 194: Anhedonia, Joylessness
Volume 195: Persistent Sadness
Volume 196: Obesity, Food Addiction
Volume 197: Parents of Abused Children
Volume 198: Letting Go and Letting Be
Volume 199: Childhood Sexual Abuse
Volume 200: Fear of Loss

www.ingramcontent.com/pod-product-compliance
Lightning Source LLC
Chambersburg PA
CBHW030501220526
45464CB00006B/2604

HYPNOTHERAPY SESSION SCRIPTS

www.ingosimon.com

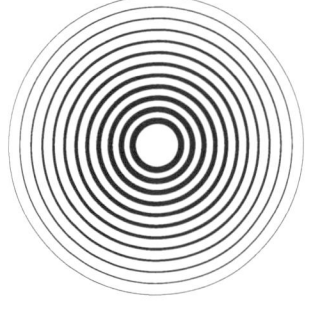

ISBN 9798334627628

Ten Hypnoses

Heart Anxiety Neurosis

39

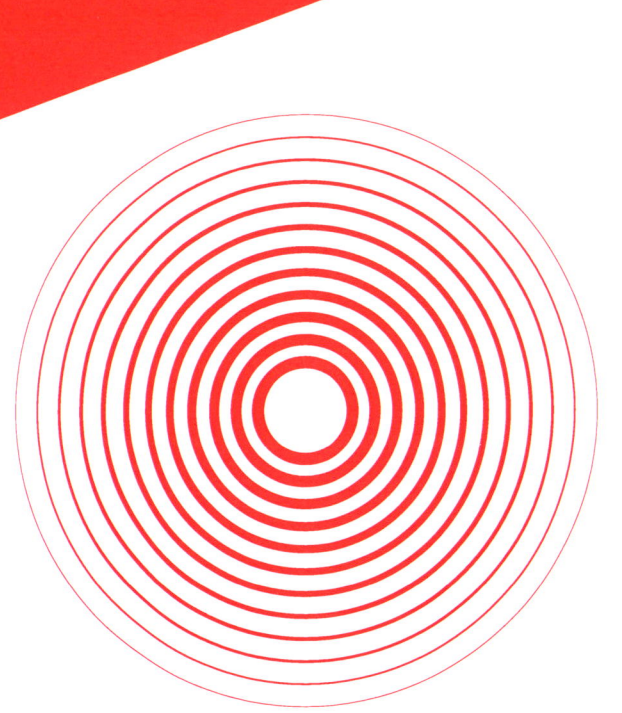

Ingo Michael Simon